This publication is intended to provide educational information for the reader on the covered subjects. It is not intended to take the place of personalized medical counseling, diagnosis, and treatment from a trained healthcare professional.

ISBN 978-1-998455-75-1 (Paperback)
ISBN 978-1-998455-76-8 (eBook)

Printed and bound in USA
Published by Loons Press

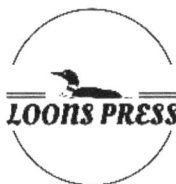

I0105932

LOONS PRESS

How To Prevent Gum Disease

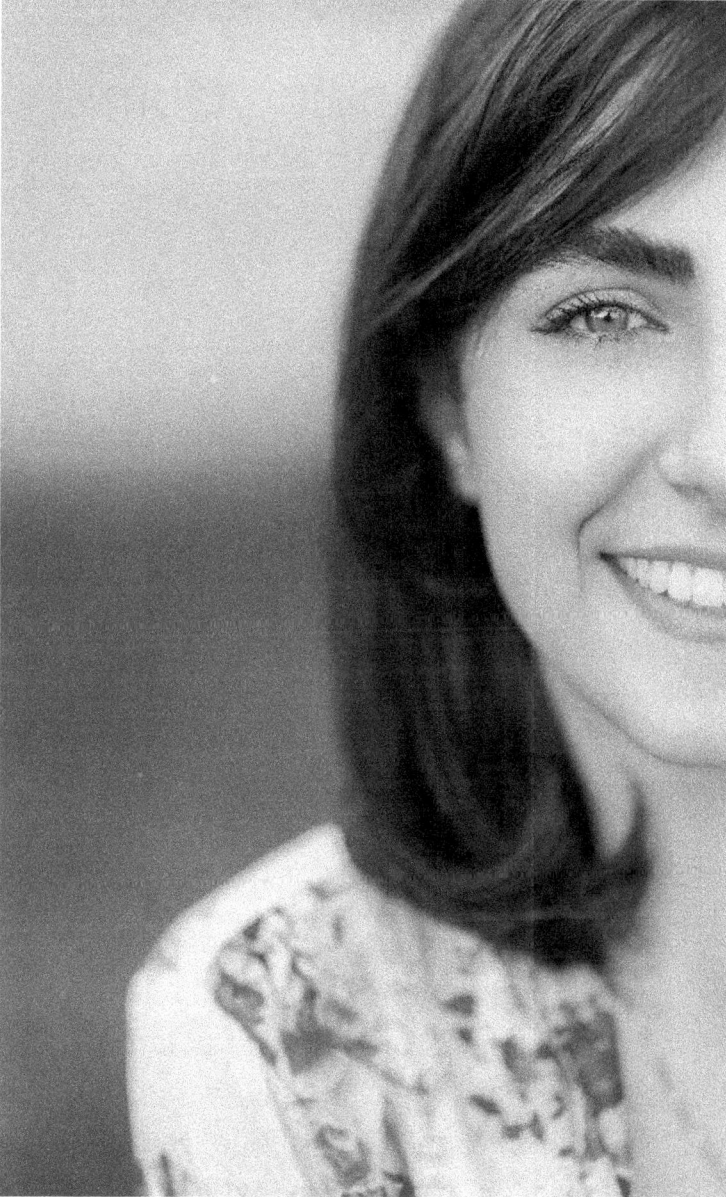

Chapter 1

Understanding Gum Disease

What is Gum Disease?

Gum disease, also known as periodontal disease, is a common condition that affects many people around the world. It is a serious infection of the gums that can lead to tooth loss if left untreated. Gum disease is caused by the buildup of plaque on the teeth, which can harden into tartar if not removed through regular brushing and flossing. This plaque and tartar can irritate the gums, causing them to become inflamed and eventually leading to gum disease.

There are two main types of gum disease: gingivitis and periodontitis. Gingivitis is the milder form of gum disease and is characterized by red, swollen gums that bleed easily when brushed or flossed. If left untreated, gingivitis can progress to periodontitis, which is a more severe form of gum disease that can lead to bone and tooth loss.

How To Prevent Gum Disease

It is important to catch gum disease early and seek treatment to prevent it from progressing to a more serious stage.

Symptoms of gum disease include red, swollen, or tender gums, bleeding when brushing or flossing, persistent bad breath, receding gums, and loose or shifting teeth. If you are experiencing any of these symptoms, it is important to see a dentist for a thorough evaluation and treatment plan. Your dentist can help you determine the best course of action to treat your gum disease and prevent it from worsening.

Preventing gum disease is key to maintaining good oral health. This includes practicing good oral hygiene habits such as brushing your teeth twice a day, flossing daily, and visiting your dentist regularly for check-ups and cleanings.

Avoiding tobacco products, eating a healthy diet, and managing stress can also help prevent gum disease. By taking care of your oral health and seeking treatment for gum disease early, you can protect your smile and overall health.

In conclusion, gum disease is a common condition that can lead to serious complications if left untreated. By understanding the causes and symptoms of gum disease, you can take steps to prevent it and maintain good oral health.

Remember to practice good oral hygiene habits, see your dentist regularly, and seek treatment if you suspect you have gum disease. With proper care and attention, you can protect your smile and prevent gum disease from impacting your overall health.

Causes of Gum Disease

Gum disease, also known as periodontal disease, is a common oral health issue that affects millions of people worldwide. Understanding the causes of gum disease is crucial in order to effectively prevent and manage this condition. There are several factors that can contribute to the development of gum disease, including poor oral hygiene, smoking, genetics, hormonal changes, and certain medical conditions.

One of the primary causes of gum disease is poor oral hygiene. Failure to brush and floss regularly allows plaque and bacteria to accumulate on the teeth and gums, leading to inflammation and infection. Plaque is a sticky film that forms on the teeth and contains harmful bacteria that can irritate the gums and cause them to become red, swollen, and tender. Over time, untreated plaque can harden into tartar, which can only be removed by a dental professional.

Smoking is another major risk factor for gum disease. Tobacco use can weaken the immune system and reduce blood flow to the gums, making it harder for the body to fight off infections. Smokers are also more likely to develop tartar buildup on their teeth, which can exacerbate gum disease. Additionally, smoking can mask the symptoms of gum disease, making it harder to detect and treat in its early stages.

Genetics can also play a role in the development of gum disease. Some people may be genetically predisposed to have weaker gum tissue or a heightened immune response to bacteria, putting them at a higher risk for developing gum disease.

If you have a family history of gum disease, it is important to be extra vigilant about your oral hygiene and schedule regular check-ups with your dentist to monitor your gum health.

Hormonal changes, such as those that occur during puberty, pregnancy, and menopause, can also increase the risk of gum disease. Fluctuations in hormone levels can make the gums more sensitive and prone to inflammation, making it easier for bacteria to cause infection. It is important for individuals experiencing hormonal changes to pay extra attention to their oral hygiene and seek professional dental care if they notice any signs of gum disease.

Certain medical conditions, such as diabetes, cardiovascular disease, and autoimmune disorders, can also increase the risk of gum disease. These conditions can compromise the body's ability to fight off infections and can affect the health of the gums and teeth. It is important for individuals with these conditions to work closely with their healthcare providers to manage their overall health and reduce their risk of developing gum disease.

By understanding the causes of gum disease and taking proactive steps to prevent it, individuals can maintain better oral health and reduce their risk of developing serious complications related to gum disease.

Symptoms of Gum Disease

Symptoms of gum disease can vary in severity and can manifest differently for each individual. One common symptom is bleeding gums, especially when brushing or flossing. This occurs because of the inflammation and irritation of the gums caused by the buildup of plaque and bacteria.

Another common symptom is swollen or tender gums, which can be uncomfortable and make it difficult to eat or speak. If left untreated, gum disease can progress to more serious symptoms such as receding gums, loose teeth, and even tooth loss.

In addition to bleeding and swollen gums, bad breath can also be a symptom of gum disease. This is often caused by the bacteria in the mouth releasing toxins that contribute to the foul odor. Persistent bad breath, also known as halitosis, can be embarrassing and affect your confidence in social situations. It is important to address this symptom by seeking treatment for gum disease to improve not only your oral health but also your overall well-being.

Another symptom of gum disease is the formation of pockets between the teeth and gums. These pockets can harbor bacteria and plaque, leading to further inflammation and infection. If left untreated, these pockets can deepen, causing the gums to recede and exposing the roots of the teeth. This can make the teeth more sensitive to hot and cold temperatures and increase the risk of tooth decay and gum infections.

In some cases, gum disease can also cause changes in the appearance of the gums, such as a change in color from pink to red or purple. This can be an indication of more advanced stages of gum disease, such as periodontitis.

Other symptoms of advanced gum disease include pus between the teeth and gums, pain when chewing, and a bad taste in the mouth. It is important to seek professional treatment if you experience any of these symptoms to prevent further damage to your oral health.

Overall, recognizing the symptoms of gum disease is crucial in preventing it from progressing to more serious stages. By paying attention to signs such as bleeding gums, bad breath, and changes in the appearance of the gums, you can take proactive steps to improve your oral health. Seeking treatment from a dental professional is essential in managing gum disease and preventing long-term complications such as tooth loss. Remember, early detection and intervention are key to maintaining a healthy smile and preventing gum disease from affecting your quality of life.

How To Prevent Gum Disease

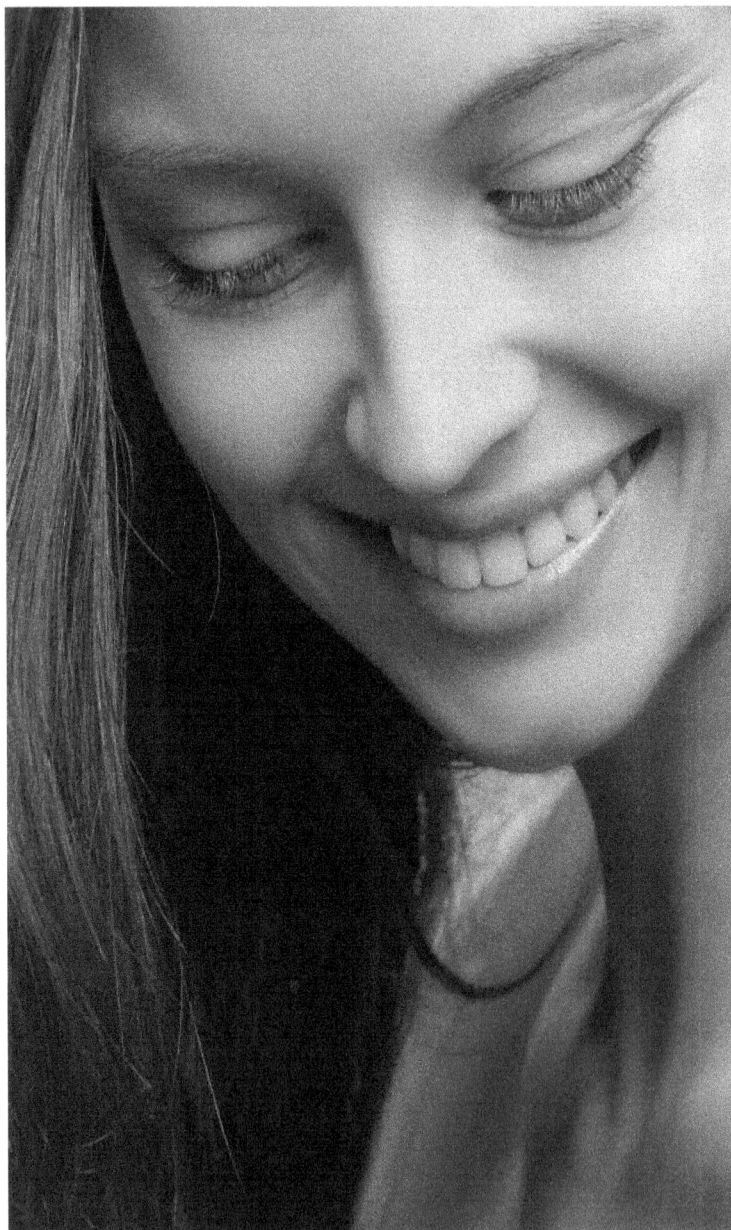

Chapter 2

Importance of Preventing Gum Disease

Effects of Untreated Gum Disease

Untreated gum disease can have serious consequences on your oral health and overall well-being. One of the most common effects of untreated gum disease is tooth loss.

As gum disease progresses, the bacteria and plaque buildup can cause the gums to pull away from the teeth, creating pockets where more bacteria can thrive. This can eventually lead to the destruction of the supporting structures of the teeth, resulting in tooth loss. Losing teeth can not only affect your ability to chew and speak properly, but it can also have a significant impact on your self-esteem and confidence.

Another effect of untreated gum disease is bad breath, also known as halitosis. The bacteria that cause gum disease release toxins that can produce a foul odor in your mouth. This can be embarrassing and can affect your social interactions.

Additionally, the toxins released by the bacteria can also enter your bloodstream and affect other parts of your body, increasing your risk for other health problems such as heart disease, diabetes, and respiratory infections.

Untreated gum disease can also lead to gum recession, where the gums pull away from the teeth and expose the roots. This can cause sensitivity to hot and cold temperatures, as well as an increased risk for tooth decay on the roots of the teeth. Additionally, gum recession can make your teeth appear longer and uneven, affecting the aesthetics of your smile. It is important to address gum recession early on to prevent further damage to your teeth and gums.

In severe cases, untreated gum disease can lead to abscesses, which are painful infections that can form at the root of a tooth or in the space between the teeth and gums. Abscesses can cause severe pain, swelling, and pus drainage, and can even lead to systemic infections if left untreated.

It is important to seek immediate dental care if you suspect you have an abscess, as it can have serious consequences on your oral and overall health.

Overall, the effects of untreated gum disease can be detrimental to your oral health and overall well-being. It is important to practice good oral hygiene habits, such as brushing and flossing regularly, visiting your dentist for regular check-ups and cleanings, and addressing any signs of gum disease early on to prevent these negative effects. Taking care of your gums is essential for maintaining a healthy smile and a healthy body.

The Link Between Gum Disease and Overall Health

Gum disease, also known as periodontal disease, is a common condition that affects the gums and bones supporting the teeth. While it may seem like a minor issue, gum disease can actually have a significant impact on your overall health. Research has shown that there is a strong link between gum disease and various health problems, including heart disease, diabetes, and respiratory diseases. This connection highlights the importance of maintaining good oral health to prevent gum disease and protect your overall well-being.

One of the main reasons why gum disease is linked to other health issues is inflammation. When bacteria build up in the mouth and cause gum disease, the body's immune response leads to inflammation in the gums. This inflammation can spread to other parts of the body, contributing to chronic inflammation and increasing the risk of developing diseases such as heart disease and diabetes. By preventing and treating gum disease, you can reduce inflammation in your body and lower your risk of developing these serious health conditions.

In addition to inflammation, gum disease can also affect your body's ability to control blood sugar levels. Research has shown that people with diabetes are more likely to have gum disease, and that untreated gum disease can make it harder to control blood sugar levels. By maintaining good oral hygiene and preventing gum disease, you can help manage your diabetes and reduce the risk of complications associated with the disease. Taking care of your oral health is an important part of managing your overall health, especially if you have diabetes.

Furthermore, gum disease has been associated with an increased risk of respiratory diseases such as pneumonia and chronic obstructive pulmonary disease (COPD). This connection is thought to be due to the bacteria in the mouth being inhaled into the lungs, leading to infections and inflammation.

By preventing gum disease and maintaining good oral health, you can reduce the risk of respiratory infections and protect your lung health. It's clear that taking care of your gums is not just about preserving your teeth – it's also about safeguarding your overall health.

In conclusion, the link between gum disease and overall health is a strong reminder of the importance of good oral hygiene. By preventing and treating gum disease, you can reduce inflammation in your body, control blood sugar levels, and protect yourself from respiratory diseases.

If you have gum disease, it's essential to work with your dentist to develop a treatment plan that addresses both your oral health and your overall well-being. With proper care and attention, you can prevent gum disease and enjoy better health for years to come.

Benefits of Preventing Gum Disease

Gum disease is a common oral health issue that affects many people around the world. However, it is important to understand the benefits of preventing gum disease in order to maintain good oral health. By taking the necessary steps to prevent gum disease, individuals can avoid the pain, discomfort, and potential complications associated with this condition.

One of the key benefits of preventing gum disease is the preservation of overall oral health. Gum disease can lead to issues such as gum recession, tooth loss, and even bone loss in severe cases. By maintaining healthy gums through proper oral hygiene practices and regular dental check-ups, individuals can prevent these issues from occurring and preserve their oral health in the long run.

Additionally, preventing gum disease can also have a positive impact on one's overall health. Research has shown that there is a strong link between gum disease and other systemic health conditions, such as heart disease, diabetes, and respiratory infections. By preventing gum disease, individuals can reduce their risk of developing these serious health issues and improve their overall well-being.

Another benefit of preventing gum disease is the potential cost savings associated with avoiding expensive dental treatments. Treating gum disease can be costly, especially if it has progressed to a more advanced stage. By taking proactive steps to prevent gum disease, individuals can avoid the need for costly treatments and save money in the long run.

Overall, the benefits of preventing gum disease are numerous and far-reaching. By maintaining good oral hygiene habits, attending regular dental check-ups, and seeking treatment at the first sign of gum disease, individuals can protect their oral health, improve their overall health, and save money on dental treatments. It is never too late to start taking steps to prevent gum disease and reap the benefits of a healthy smile.

How To Prevent Gum Disease

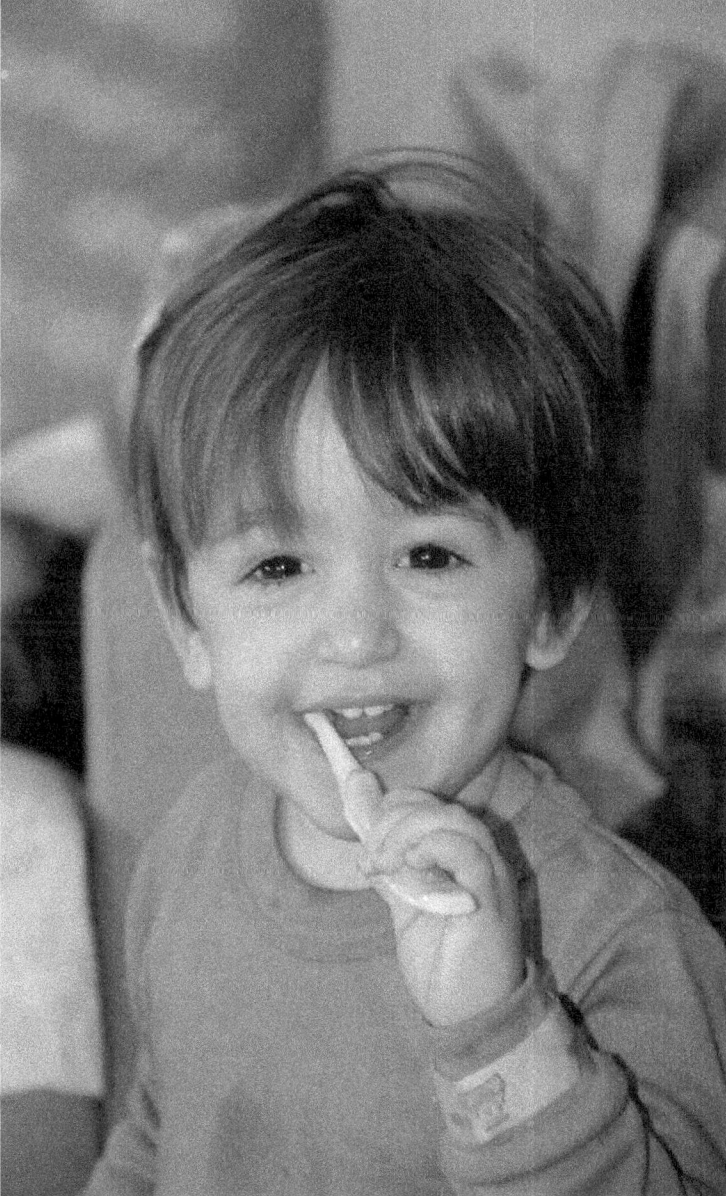

Chapter 3

Daily Oral Hygiene Practices

Brushing Techniques for Healthy Gums

In order to prevent gum disease and maintain healthy gums, it is crucial to follow proper brushing techniques. Brushing your teeth is an essential part of your oral hygiene routine, and when done correctly, it can help prevent plaque buildup and gum disease. Here are some brushing techniques that can help you achieve healthier gums.

First and foremost, it is important to choose the right toothbrush. Opt for a soft-bristled toothbrush that is gentle on your gums. Hard-bristled brushes can cause damage to the gums and lead to irritation. Additionally, consider using an electric toothbrush, as they are more effective at removing plaque and bacteria from the gum line.

How To Prevent Gum Disease

When brushing your teeth, be sure to brush gently and in a circular motion. Avoid using too much force, as this can cause damage to your gums. Focus on brushing each tooth individually, making sure to reach all surfaces, including the front, back, and chewing surfaces. Pay special attention to the gum line, as this is where plaque tends to accumulate.

It is recommended to brush your teeth at least twice a day, for two minutes each time. This ensures that you are effectively removing plaque and bacteria from your teeth and gums. Additionally, be sure to replace your toothbrush every three to four months, or sooner if the bristles are frayed.

In addition to proper brushing techniques, it is important to floss daily to remove plaque and food particles from between your teeth. This helps prevent gum disease and promotes healthy gums. Consider using an antimicrobial mouthwash as well, to help kill bacteria and reduce plaque buildup.

By following these brushing techniques and incorporating them into your daily oral hygiene routine, you can help prevent gum disease and maintain healthy gums. Remember, taking care of your gums is an essential part of maintaining good oral health and overall wellbeing.

Importance of Flossing

Flossing is an essential part of maintaining good oral health and preventing gum disease. Many people underestimate the importance of flossing, but it plays a crucial role in removing plaque and bacteria from between teeth and along the gumline. Failure to floss regularly can lead to the buildup of plaque, which can eventually harden into tartar and cause gum disease.

By incorporating flossing into your daily oral hygiene routine, you can significantly reduce your risk of developing gum disease and other oral health problems.

How To Prevent Gum Disease

One of the main reasons why flossing is so important for preventing gum disease is that it helps to remove food particles and plaque from hard-to-reach areas that your toothbrush can't reach. When left unchecked, plaque can irritate the gums and lead to inflammation, swelling, and bleeding. Over time, this can progress into gingivitis and eventually periodontitis if not properly treated. Flossing helps to prevent the buildup of plaque and reduces the risk of gum disease by keeping your teeth and gums clean and healthy.

In addition to removing plaque and bacteria from between teeth, flossing also helps to stimulate the gums and improve circulation in the gum tissue. This can help to strengthen the gums and make them more resistant to infection and disease.

By flossing regularly, you can promote better gum health and reduce your risk of developing gum disease. It is recommended to floss at least once a day, preferably before brushing your teeth, to ensure that you are effectively removing plaque and debris from between your teeth and along the gumline.

For people who already have gum disease, flossing is even more important to prevent further progression of the disease. Regular flossing can help to remove plaque and bacteria from the pockets that have formed between the teeth and gums, reducing inflammation and promoting healing. In combination with other treatments prescribed by your dentist, flossing can play a crucial role in managing and treating gum disease. By incorporating flossing into your daily routine, you can take control of your oral health and prevent gum disease from worsening.

Overall, flossing is a simple yet effective way to prevent gum disease and maintain good oral health. By taking a few minutes each day to floss your teeth, you can remove plaque and bacteria from hard-to-reach areas and reduce your risk of developing gum disease.

Whether you are looking to prevent gum disease or manage existing gum disease, flossing is a key component of a comprehensive oral hygiene routine. Make flossing a priority in your daily routine and enjoy the benefits of healthier teeth and gums for years to come.

Using Mouthwash to Prevent Gum Disease

Using mouthwash is an important step in preventing gum disease. Gum disease, also known as periodontal disease, is a common condition that can lead to serious oral health issues if left untreated. By incorporating mouthwash into your daily oral hygiene routine, you can help reduce the buildup of plaque and bacteria in your mouth, which are major contributors to gum disease.

Choosing the right mouthwash is key to effectively preventing gum disease. Look for a mouthwash that is specifically designed to fight bacteria and plaque, as these are the main culprits behind gum disease. Some mouthwashes also contain ingredients like fluoride or essential oils that can further help to protect your gums and teeth.

It's important to read the label and choose a mouthwash that is approved by the American Dental Association (ADA) for its effectiveness in preventing gum disease.

To use mouthwash effectively in preventing gum disease, it's important to incorporate it into your daily oral hygiene routine. After brushing and flossing your teeth, rinse with a mouthwash for at least 30 seconds, making sure to swish it around your mouth thoroughly. This will help to kill bacteria and plaque that may linger in hard-to-reach areas of your mouth, further reducing your risk of developing gum disease.

In addition to using mouthwash, it's important to maintain good oral hygiene habits to prevent gum disease. This includes brushing your teeth at least twice a day, flossing daily, and visiting your dentist regularly for check-ups and cleanings.

By combining the use of mouthwash with these other oral hygiene practices, you can significantly reduce your risk of developing gum disease and maintain a healthy smile for years to come.

In conclusion, using mouthwash is an effective way to prevent gum disease and maintain good oral health. By choosing the right mouthwash, incorporating it into your daily routine, and maintaining good oral hygiene habits, you can reduce your risk of developing gum disease and enjoy a healthy smile. Remember to consult with your dentist for personalized recommendations on the best mouthwash for your specific oral health needs.

How To Prevent Gum Disease

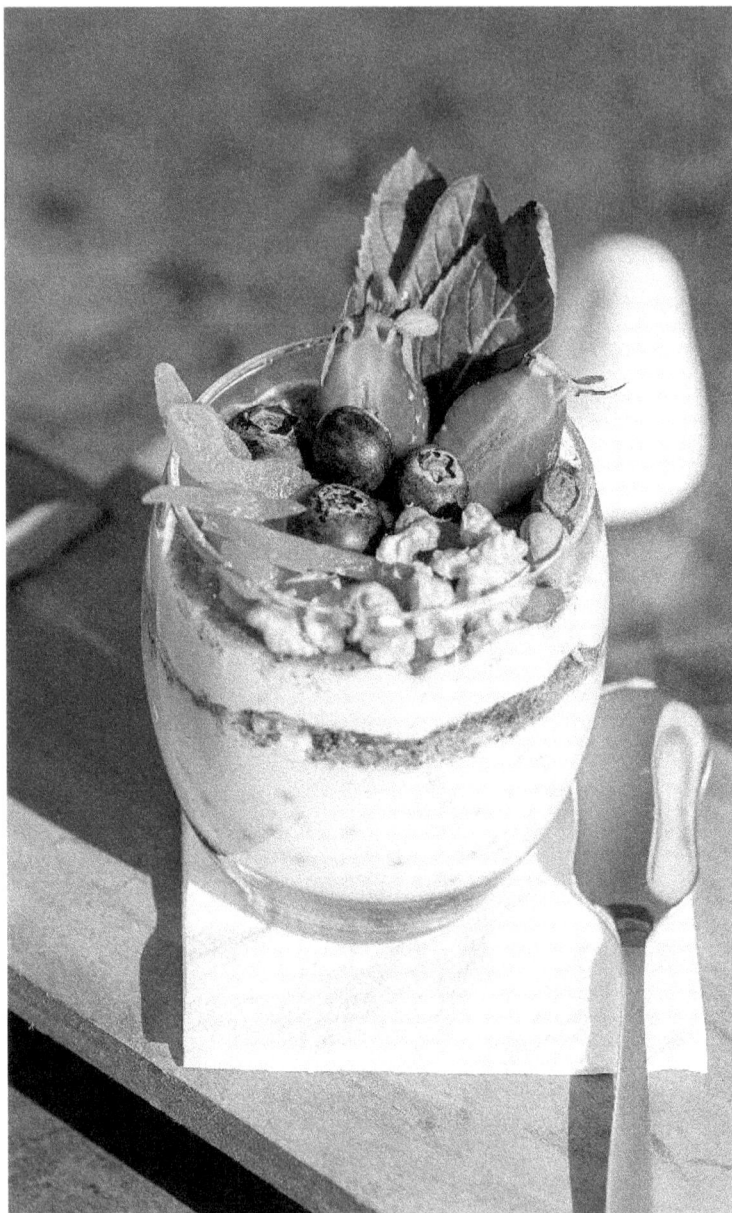

Chapter 4

Nutrition and Gum Health

Foods That Promote Healthy Gums

Gum disease is a common oral health issue that affects many people. One of the keys to preventing gum disease is maintaining healthy gums through proper nutrition. In this subchapter, we will discuss foods that promote healthy gums and help prevent gum disease.

One food that is particularly beneficial for gum health is leafy greens. Greens such as spinach, kale, and Swiss chard are rich in vitamins and minerals that are essential for healthy gums. These foods are also high in fiber, which can help remove plaque and bacteria from the teeth and gums.

Another food that can promote healthy gums is yogurt. Yogurt contains probiotics, which are beneficial bacteria that can help maintain a healthy balance of bacteria in the mouth. This can help prevent the growth of harmful bacteria that can lead to gum disease.

Berries, such as strawberries, blueberries, and raspberries, are also great for gum health. Berries are packed with antioxidants, which can help reduce inflammation in the gums and prevent gum disease. They are also low in sugar, which can help prevent cavities and gum disease.

Nuts and seeds are another important food group for promoting healthy gums. Nuts and seeds are high in nutrients such as vitamin E, which can help reduce inflammation in the gums. They are also high in fiber, which can help remove plaque and bacteria from the teeth and gums.

Incorporating these foods into your diet can help promote healthy gums and prevent gum disease. By eating a balanced diet rich in leafy greens, yogurt, berries, nuts, and seeds, you can help maintain optimal gum health and reduce your risk of developing gum disease. Remember, prevention is key when it comes to gum disease, so be sure to prioritize your oral health by eating foods that promote healthy gums.

Foods to Avoid for Gum Health

In order to maintain healthy gums and prevent gum disease, it is important to be mindful of the foods we consume on a daily basis. Some foods can actually contribute to the development and progression of gum disease, so it is crucial to be aware of which foods to avoid for optimal gum health.

One of the main culprits when it comes to worsening gum health is sugary foods and beverages. Consuming too much sugar can lead to the buildup of plaque on the teeth, which can eventually cause gum inflammation and disease. It is best to limit the intake of sugary treats such as candies, sodas, and sweetened snacks to protect your gums from harm.

Another type of food to steer clear of for gum health is acidic foods and drinks. Acidic foods can erode the enamel on your teeth, making them more susceptible to gum disease. Citrus fruits, vinegar-based dressings, and carbonated beverages are examples of acidic foods that should be consumed in moderation to prevent gum issues.

Foods that are high in carbohydrates, such as white bread, pasta, and crackers, can also negatively impact your gum health. Carbohydrates break down into sugars in the mouth, providing fuel for harmful bacteria to thrive and cause gum disease. Opt for whole grain alternatives instead to protect your gums and overall oral health.

Lastly, it is important to avoid sticky and hard foods that can damage your gums and teeth. Sticky candies, chewy snacks, and hard nuts can all contribute to gum irritation and even lead to gum recession. Be mindful of the texture of the foods you eat and opt for softer options to protect your gums from unnecessary harm.

By being aware of the foods to avoid for gum health and making conscious choices in your diet, you can greatly reduce your risk of developing gum disease and maintain a healthy smile for years to come. Remember to also practice good oral hygiene habits, such as brushing and flossing regularly, to further protect your gums and overall oral health.

Importance of Water for Gum Health

As individuals who are struggling with gum disease, it is crucial to understand the importance of water for gum health. Water plays a vital role in maintaining good oral health, including keeping your gums healthy and preventing gum disease. Staying hydrated by drinking an adequate amount of water each day can help wash away bacteria and food particles that can contribute to gum disease. Additionally, water helps stimulate saliva production, which is essential for neutralizing acids and protecting your teeth and gums.

One of the key benefits of water for gum health is its ability to help keep your mouth clean. Water can rinse away bacteria and food particles that can accumulate in the mouth and lead to gum disease. By drinking water throughout the day, you can help prevent plaque buildup and reduce the risk of developing gum disease.

Additionally, water can help freshen your breath and reduce the likelihood of developing bad breath, another common symptom of gum disease.

In addition to helping keep your mouth clean, water can also help promote healthy gums by keeping them hydrated. Dry mouth can be a contributing factor to gum disease, as saliva plays a crucial role in protecting your teeth and gums. By staying hydrated with water, you can help prevent dry mouth and ensure that your gums remain healthy and well-hydrated. This can help reduce inflammation and discomfort associated with gum disease and promote overall gum health.

Furthermore, drinking water can help promote overall health and well-being, which can have a positive impact on your gum health. Staying hydrated with water can help boost your immune system, which plays a crucial role in fighting off infections and preventing gum disease. Additionally, water can help improve digestion and nutrient absorption, which can contribute to overall oral health. By incorporating more water into your daily routine, you can help support your body's natural defenses against gum disease and promote optimal gum health.

In conclusion, water is a simple yet powerful tool for maintaining good gum health and preventing gum disease. By staying hydrated with water throughout the day, you can help wash away bacteria, keep your gums hydrated, and promote overall health and well-being. Make sure to drink an adequate amount of water each day and incorporate it into your oral care routine to help protect your gums and prevent gum disease. Remember, a well-hydrated mouth is a healthy mouth!

How To Prevent Gum Disease

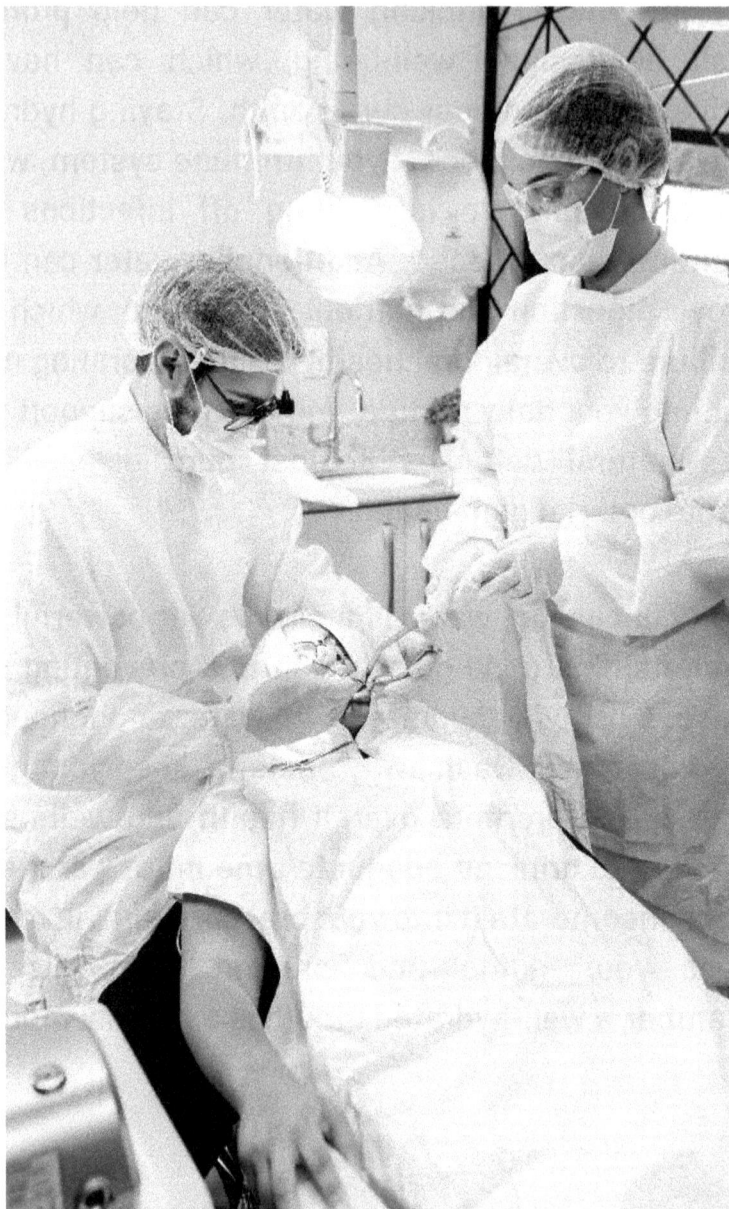

A Complete Guide for Better Oral Health

Chapter 5

Regular Dental Check-ups

Importance of Dental Cleanings

Regular dental cleanings are essential for preventing and treating gum disease. Gum disease is a common condition that affects millions of people worldwide. It is caused by the buildup of plaque and tartar on the teeth, which can lead to inflammation and infection of the gums. Without proper treatment, gum disease can progress to more serious conditions, such as periodontitis, which can cause tooth loss and other complications.

Dental cleanings are important because they help remove plaque and tartar from the teeth and gums, reducing the risk of gum disease. During a dental cleaning, a dental hygienist will use special tools to remove plaque and tartar from the teeth and gums, as well as polish the teeth to remove stains and improve their appearance. Regular dental cleanings can also help prevent bad breath, tooth decay, and other oral health problems.

In addition to removing plaque and tartar, dental cleanings also allow your dentist to check for signs of gum disease and other oral health issues. Your dentist will examine your teeth and gums for signs of inflammation, bleeding, and other symptoms of gum disease. If gum disease is detected, your dentist can recommend appropriate treatment to help prevent further damage to your gums and teeth.

It is recommended that people with gum disease schedule regular dental cleanings every six months to maintain good oral health and prevent gum disease from progressing. In some cases, your dentist may recommend more frequent cleanings, depending on the severity of your gum disease. By staying on top of your dental cleanings, you can help prevent gum disease and keep your teeth and gums healthy for years to come.

Overall, dental cleanings play a crucial role in preventing gum disease and maintaining good oral health. By removing plaque and tartar from the teeth and gums, dental cleanings help reduce the risk of gum disease and other oral health problems.

If you have gum disease, it is important to schedule regular dental cleanings to prevent further damage to your gums and teeth. Talk to your dentist about the importance of dental cleanings and how they can help you maintain a healthy smile.

Monitoring Gum Health with Regular Check-ups

Regular check-ups with your dentist are crucial in monitoring the health of your gums. By scheduling routine appointments, your dentist can keep track of any changes in your gum health and address any issues before they progress. During these check-ups, your dentist will examine your gums for signs of inflammation, bleeding, or recession, which are all indicators of gum disease.

By catching these warning signs early, you can prevent gum disease from advancing and causing more serious complications.

In addition to monitoring the health of your gums, regular check-ups also allow your dentist to provide professional cleanings to remove plaque and tartar buildup. Plaque is a sticky film of bacteria that forms on your teeth and gums, and if not removed regularly, it can harden into tartar, which can only be removed by a dental professional. By keeping your teeth and gums clean, you can reduce your risk of developing gum disease and other oral health problems.

During your check-ups, your dentist may also recommend additional preventive measures to help maintain the health of your gums. This may include using a prescription mouthwash or dental floss specifically designed to target gum disease. Your dentist may also provide tips on proper oral hygiene techniques, such as brushing and flossing, to help prevent gum disease from developing or progressing.

By staying on top of your gum health with regular check-ups, you can take proactive steps to prevent gum disease and maintain a healthy smile. Remember that prevention is key when it comes to gum disease, and early detection and treatment are essential in preserving your oral health.

So, make sure to schedule regular check-ups with your dentist and follow their recommendations to keep your gums healthy and disease-free. Your smile will thank you for it!

Treatment Options for Gum Disease

If you have been diagnosed with gum disease, it is important to explore your treatment options to prevent further damage to your oral health. There are several effective treatments available that can help manage and even reverse the effects of gum disease. In this subchapter, we will discuss some of the most common treatment options for gum disease and how they can help improve your oral health.

One of the most common treatments for gum disease is scaling and root planing. This procedure involves deep cleaning of the teeth and gums to remove plaque and tartar buildup that can contribute to gum disease.

During scaling, your dentist will use special tools to remove plaque and tartar from the surface of your teeth and below the gumline. Root planing involves smoothing out the roots of the teeth to prevent bacteria from reattaching and causing further damage. This procedure can help reduce inflammation and promote healing of the gums.

Another treatment option for gum disease is antibiotic therapy. In some cases, your dentist may prescribe antibiotics to help kill the bacteria causing the infection in your gums. This can help reduce inflammation and promote healing of the gums. Antibiotic therapy may be prescribed in the form of a mouth rinse, gel, or oral medication, depending on the severity of your gum disease.

In more severe cases of gum disease, surgery may be necessary to effectively treat the infection. Gum surgery can help remove damaged tissue, reduce pockets around the teeth, and promote healing of the gums. There are several types of gum surgery available, including flap surgery, bone grafts, and tissue regeneration procedures. Your dentist will work with you to determine the best surgical option for your specific needs.

In addition to professional treatments, it is important to maintain good oral hygiene habits at home to prevent gum disease from recurring. This includes brushing your teeth twice a day, flossing daily, and using an antiseptic mouthwash to help kill bacteria in your mouth. It is also important to attend regular dental check-ups and cleanings to monitor the health of your gums and prevent any further damage. By following these treatment options and practicing good oral hygiene, you can help prevent gum disease and maintain a healthy smile for years to come.

How To Prevent Gum Disease

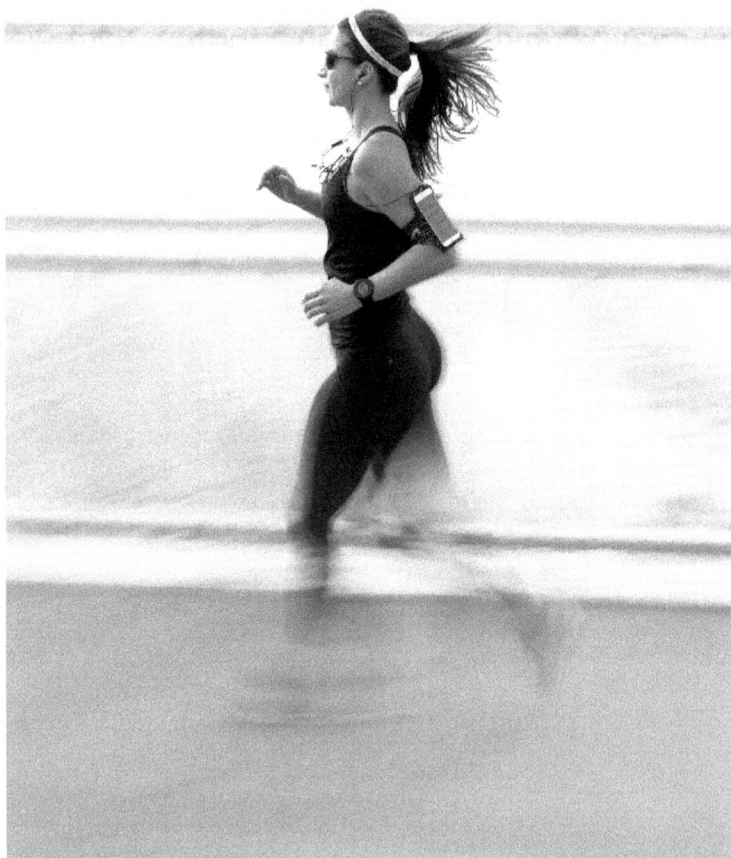

Chapter 6

Lifestyle Habits That Affect Gum Health

The Impact of Smoking on Gum Disease

Smoking has a significant impact on gum disease, as it is a major risk factor for developing periodontal disease. Research has shown that smokers are more likely to experience gum inflammation, bleeding, and bone loss compared to non-smokers. The chemicals in cigarettes can weaken the immune system, making it harder for the body to fight off infections in the mouth, leading to the progression of gum disease.

Furthermore, smoking can also mask the symptoms of gum disease, making it harder to detect and treat in its early stages. This delay in diagnosis can result in more severe damage to the gums and bone structure, ultimately leading to tooth loss. It is important for individuals with gum disease who smoke to be aware of these risks and take proactive steps to improve their oral health.

Quitting smoking is one of the most effective ways to prevent gum disease and improve overall oral health. By eliminating smoking from your daily routine, you can reduce inflammation in the gums, improve blood flow to the mouth, and enhance the body's ability to heal and repair damaged tissues. This can help to slow down the progression of gum disease and prevent further complications.

In addition to quitting smoking, individuals with gum disease can also benefit from practicing good oral hygiene habits. This includes brushing and flossing regularly, using an antiseptic mouthwash, and visiting the dentist for regular check-ups and cleanings. By maintaining a clean and healthy mouth, you can reduce the risk of developing gum disease and improve the overall health of your teeth and gums.

Overall, the impact of smoking on gum disease is significant and can have serious consequences for oral health. By quitting smoking and adopting a comprehensive oral care routine, individuals with gum disease can take control of their oral health and prevent further damage to their gums and teeth.

It is never too late to make positive changes for better oral health, and taking steps to quit smoking and improve oral hygiene can make a significant difference in preventing gum disease.

Stress Management for Better Oral Health

Living with gum disease can be a stressful experience. The constant worry about your oral health, the pain and discomfort, and the financial burden of treatment can take a toll on your mental wellbeing. However, stress can also have a direct impact on your oral health, exacerbating the symptoms of gum disease and making it harder to manage. That's why learning how to effectively manage stress is crucial for maintaining good oral health.

One of the ways that stress can negatively affect your oral health is by weakening your immune system. When you are stressed, your body produces more of the hormone cortisol, which can suppress the immune system and make it harder for your body to fight off infections, including gum disease.

This can lead to an increase in inflammation and bacteria in your mouth, making it more difficult to control the progression of gum disease.

In addition to weakening your immune system, stress can also lead to unhealthy habits that can further exacerbate gum disease. For example, many people turn to unhealthy coping mechanisms like smoking, drinking alcohol, or indulging in sugary snacks when they are stressed. These habits can increase the risk of gum disease and other oral health issues, making it even more important to find healthier ways to manage stress.

Fortunately, there are many effective strategies for managing stress that can help improve your oral health. Regular exercise, meditation, deep breathing exercises, and spending time in nature are all great ways to reduce stress and promote overall wellbeing. It's also important to prioritize self-care and make time for activities that bring you joy and relaxation, whether it's reading a book, taking a bath, or spending time with loved ones.

By taking steps to manage your stress effectively, you can not only improve your mental wellbeing but also support better oral health. Remember, stress is a natural part of life, but it doesn't have to control you. By incorporating stress management techniques into your daily routine, you can take control of your oral health and prevent gum disease from worsening.

Exercise and Gum Disease Prevention

Exercise plays a crucial role in preventing gum disease. Regular physical activity can help improve overall health and boost the immune system, making it easier for the body to fight off infections, including gum disease. When you exercise, you increase blood flow throughout the body, including to the gums, which can help reduce inflammation and promote healing. Additionally, exercise can help reduce stress, which is a known risk factor for gum disease.

How To Prevent Gum Disease

Incorporating a combination of aerobic exercise, strength training, and flexibility exercises into your routine can help improve your overall health and reduce your risk of developing gum disease. Aerobic exercises, such as walking, jogging, or cycling, can help improve circulation and reduce inflammation in the gums.

Strength training exercises, like weightlifting or bodyweight exercises, can help build muscle and improve immune function. Flexibility exercises, such as yoga or stretching, can help improve range of motion and reduce tension in the body, which can also benefit your oral health.

It's important to note that while exercise can help prevent gum disease, it is not a replacement for good oral hygiene practices. Brushing your teeth twice a day, flossing daily, and visiting your dentist regularly are all essential for maintaining healthy gums. However, adding exercise to your routine can further enhance your oral health and overall well-being.

If you have gum disease, incorporating exercise into your daily routine can help improve your oral health and prevent further progression of the disease. Talk to your dentist or healthcare provider about the best types of exercise for your specific situation. They may be able to provide recommendations based on your individual needs and limitations.

In conclusion, exercise is a powerful tool for preventing gum disease. By incorporating regular physical activity into your routine, you can improve circulation, boost your immune system, and reduce inflammation in the gums.

Remember to also practice good oral hygiene habits and visit your dentist regularly for check-ups and cleanings to maintain healthy gums. With a comprehensive approach to oral health that includes exercise, you can take control of your gum disease and prevent further complications in the future.

How To Prevent Gum Disease

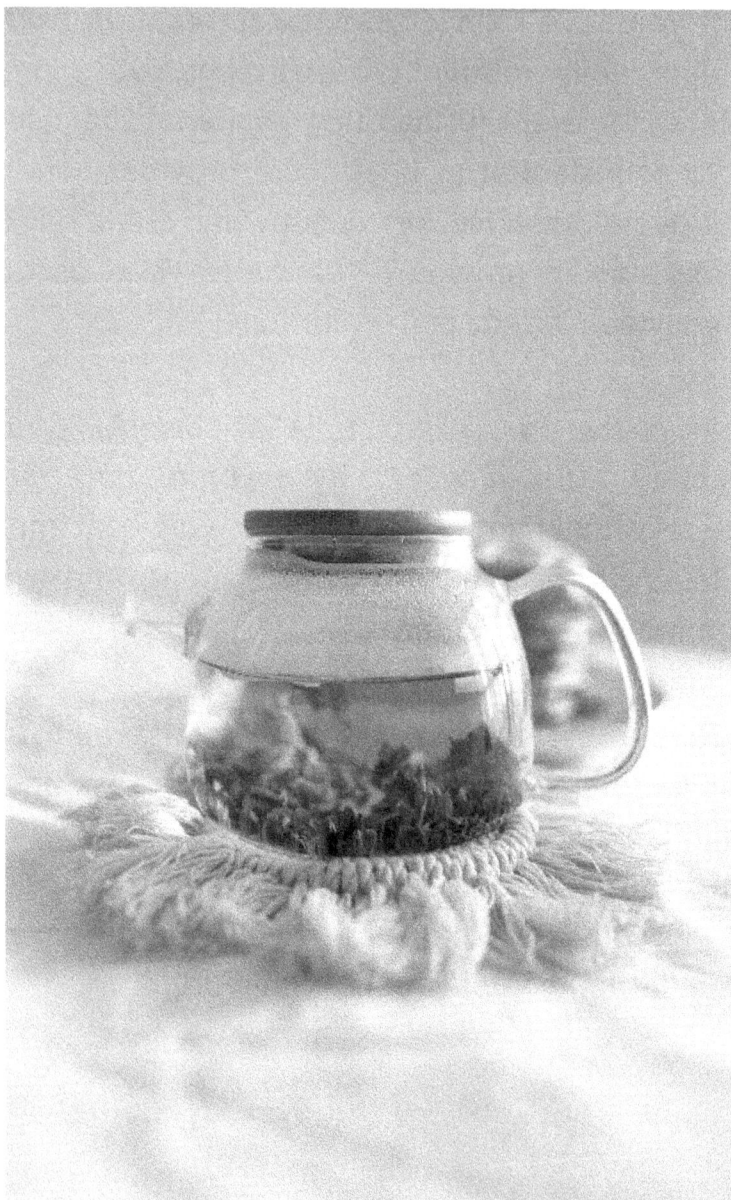

Chapter 7

Home Remedies for Gum Health

Oil Pulling for Gum Health

Oil pulling is an ancient Ayurvedic practice that involves swishing oil around in your mouth for a period of time to improve oral health. This technique has gained popularity in recent years as a natural remedy for gum disease. Oil pulling can help reduce inflammation in the gums, remove harmful bacteria, and promote overall gum health.

One of the most common oils used for oil pulling is coconut oil, due to its antimicrobial and anti-inflammatory properties. To practice oil pulling for gum health, simply take a tablespoon of coconut oil and swish it around in your mouth for 15-20 minutes each day. Make sure not to swallow the oil, as it will contain harmful bacteria and toxins that have been removed from your mouth.

Oil pulling can be a great addition to your oral hygiene routine if you have gum disease. It can help reduce the severity of gum inflammation, prevent plaque buildup, and improve overall gum health. However, oil pulling should not be used as a substitute for regular brushing and flossing. It is important to continue practicing good oral hygiene habits in addition to oil pulling for the best results.

When incorporating oil pulling into your routine, it is important to be consistent and patient. It may take some time to see noticeable improvements in your gum health, so don't get discouraged if you don't see immediate results. Remember that prevention is key when it comes to gum disease, so it is important to take proactive steps to maintain healthy gums.

Overall, oil pulling can be a beneficial practice for those looking to prevent or manage gum disease. By incorporating this ancient technique into your daily routine, you can help improve your gum health and reduce the risk of developing more serious oral health issues in the future. Give oil pulling a try and see the positive impact it can have on your gum health.

Using Natural Remedies for Gum Disease Prevention

Using natural remedies for gum disease prevention can be an effective and gentle way to maintain healthy gums. One of the most popular natural remedies is oil pulling, which involves swishing a tablespoon of coconut oil around in your mouth for 15-20 minutes each day. This practice can help reduce bacteria in the mouth and improve gum health over time.

Another natural remedy for gum disease prevention is green tea. Green tea contains antioxidants and anti-inflammatory properties that can help reduce inflammation in the gums and promote overall oral health. Drinking a cup of green tea each day can be a simple a way to support gum health.

Turmeric is another natural remedy that can be beneficial for preventing gum disease. Turmeric contains curcumin, a compound with powerful anti-inflammatory and antibacterial properties. Adding turmeric to your diet or using a turmeric mouthwash can help reduce inflammation in the gums and fight off harmful bacteria.

In addition to these natural remedies, maintaining good oral hygiene practices is essential for preventing gum disease. This includes brushing your teeth twice a day, flossing daily, and using an antibacterial mouthwash. Regular dental check-ups and cleanings are also important for monitoring and maintaining gum health.

Overall, incorporating natural remedies into your oral care routine can be a gentle and effective way to prevent gum disease. By combining these natural remedies with good oral hygiene practices, you can support healthy gums and overall oral health for years to come. Remember to consult with your dentist before trying any new natural remedies to ensure they are safe and appropriate for your individual needs.

Herbal Supplements for Gum Health

Herbal supplements have been used for centuries to promote overall health and wellness, and they can also be beneficial for improving gum health. There are several herbal supplements that have been shown to help prevent and treat gum disease.

One popular herbal supplement for gum health is tea tree oil. This essential oil has powerful antibacterial and anti-inflammatory properties that can help reduce inflammation and fight off harmful bacteria in the mouth. By adding a few drops of tea tree oil to your toothpaste or mouthwash, you can help keep your gums healthy and prevent gum disease.

Another herbal supplement that can help improve gum health is aloe vera. Aloe vera has natural anti-inflammatory and antimicrobial properties that can help reduce swelling and fight off bacteria in the mouth. You can find aloe vera in gel form at most health food stores, or you can use aloe vera juice as a mouthwash to help soothe irritated gums and promote healing.

Peppermint oil is another herbal supplement that can be beneficial for gum health. Peppermint oil has antiseptic properties that can help kill bacteria in the mouth and freshen breath. By adding a few drops of peppermint oil to your toothpaste or mouthwash, you can help keep your gums healthy and prevent gum disease.

How To Prevent Gum Disease

In addition to these herbal supplements, it is important to maintain good oral hygiene practices to prevent gum disease. This includes brushing and flossing regularly, using a fluoride toothpaste, and visiting your dentist for regular check-ups and cleanings. By incorporating herbal supplements into your oral care routine and practicing good oral hygiene, you can help prevent gum disease and keep your gums healthy for years to come.

How To Prevent Gum Disease

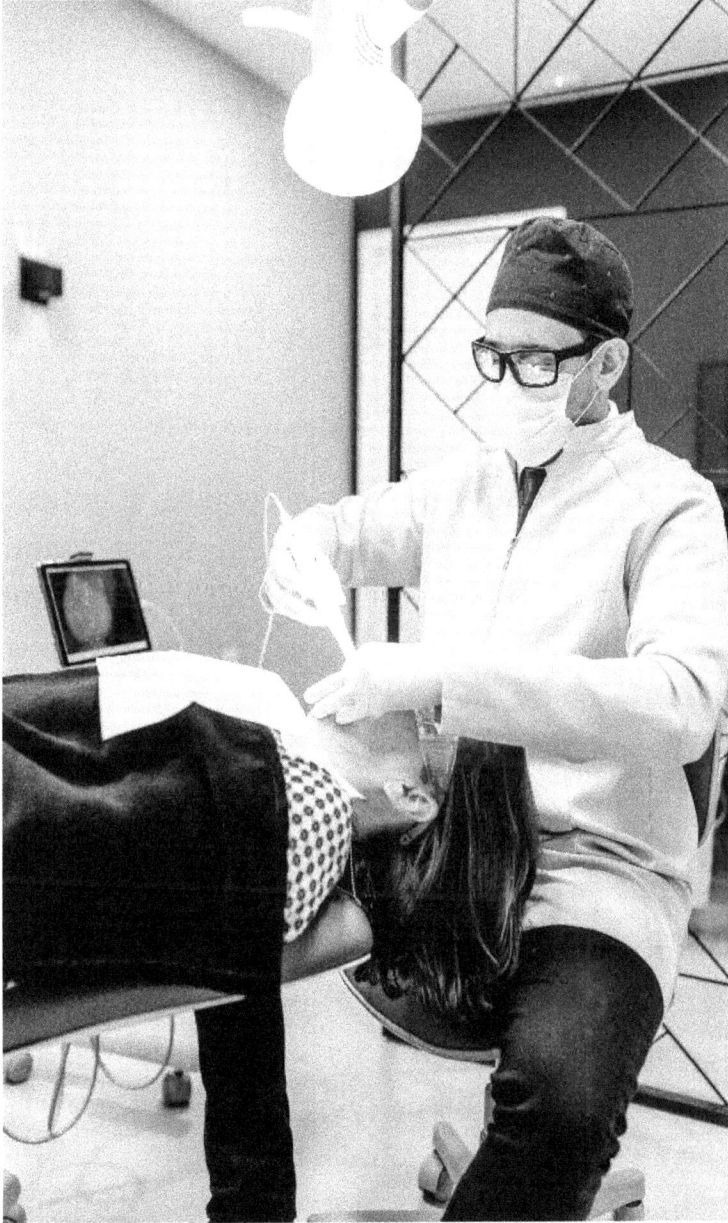

Chapter 8

Maintaining Good Oral Health Habits

Creating a Routine for Oral Hygiene

Creating a routine for oral hygiene is crucial for people who have gum disease. It is important to establish good habits that can help prevent further damage and improve overall oral health. By following a consistent routine, individuals can effectively manage their gum disease and reduce the risk of complications.

The first step in creating a routine for oral hygiene is to brush your teeth at least twice a day. Use a soft-bristled toothbrush and fluoride toothpaste to gently clean your teeth and gums. Be sure to brush for at least two minutes each time, paying close attention to the gumline where plaque tends to accumulate. Proper brushing technique is essential for removing plaque and preventing gum disease.

How To Prevent Gum Disease

In addition to brushing, it is important to floss daily to remove plaque and food particles from between your teeth. Flossing helps to prevent gum disease by removing bacteria and debris that can contribute to inflammation and infection. Use a gentle sawing motion to slide the floss between your teeth, being careful not to snap or force it into place. Flossing should be done before brushing to ensure a thorough clean.

Another important aspect of oral hygiene is using an antimicrobial mouthwash to help reduce bacteria in the mouth. Mouthwash can reach areas that brushing and flossing may miss, providing additional protection against gum disease. Choose a mouthwash that is alcohol-free and specifically formulated for gum health to maximize its benefits. Incorporating mouthwash into your daily routine can help maintain a healthy balance of bacteria in the mouth.

Lastly, regular dental check-ups and cleanings are essential for preventing gum disease and maintaining good oral health. Dentists can identify early signs of gum disease and provide treatment to prevent further progression.

Professional cleanings remove plaque and tartar buildup that cannot be removed with regular brushing and flossing. By following these tips and creating a routine for oral hygiene, individuals with gum disease can effectively manage their condition and improve their overall oral health.

Tracking Progress in Preventing Gum Disease

Tracking progress in preventing gum disease is an essential aspect of maintaining good oral health. For people who have gum disease, monitoring the effectiveness of their prevention efforts is crucial in order to prevent further damage and improve their overall oral health. By tracking progress, individuals can identify any areas of concern and make necessary adjustments to their oral hygiene routine.

One way to track progress in preventing gum disease is to regularly monitor the condition of your gums. This can be done by checking for any signs of inflammation, bleeding, or sensitivity. By keeping a close eye on the state of your gums, you can quickly identify any changes or worsening symptoms, allowing you to take immediate action to address the issue.

Another important aspect of tracking progress in preventing gum disease is to keep track of your oral hygiene habits. This includes monitoring your brushing and flossing routine, as well as any other oral hygiene practices you may be implementing. By keeping a record of your oral hygiene habits, you can identify any areas where you may be falling short and make necessary adjustments to improve your oral health.

In addition to monitoring your gums and oral hygiene habits, it is also important to keep track of any professional treatments or interventions you may be undergoing to prevent gum disease. This can include regular dental check-ups, cleanings, or treatments for gum disease. By tracking these interventions, you can ensure that you are receiving the appropriate care and that your efforts to prevent gum disease are effective.

Overall, tracking progress in preventing gum disease is essential for individuals who have gum disease. By monitoring the condition of your gums, tracking your oral hygiene habits, and keeping track of any professional treatments, you can ensure that you are taking the necessary steps to prevent further damage and improve your oral health.

By staying vigilant and proactive in tracking your progress, you can effectively prevent gum disease and maintain a healthy smile for years to come.

Seeking Professional Help When Needed

Seeking professional help when needed is crucial for individuals who have gum disease. While there are steps that can be taken at home to improve oral health, it is important to recognize when it is time to seek help from a dental professional. Gum disease is a serious condition that can lead to more severe health issues if left untreated. Therefore, it is essential to schedule regular check-ups with your dentist to monitor the health of your gums and address any concerns that may arise.

Dental professionals have the knowledge and expertise to properly diagnose and treat gum disease. They can provide personalized treatment plans based on the severity of your condition and help you take the necessary steps to improve your oral health.

Whether it is through deep cleanings, medication, or surgical procedures, dentists can offer a range of treatments to help manage and prevent gum disease from progressing.

In addition to providing treatment, dental professionals can also offer valuable advice on how to prevent gum disease in the future. They can educate patients on proper oral hygiene practices, including brushing and flossing techniques, as well as the importance of regular dental cleanings. By following their recommendations, individuals can reduce their risk of developing gum disease and maintain optimal oral health.

It is important for individuals with gum disease to not only seek professional help but also to follow through with their recommended treatment plan. Consistency is key when it comes to managing gum disease, and regular visits to the dentist can help track progress and make necessary adjustments to the treatment plan. By taking an active role in their oral health, individuals can improve their overall wellbeing and reduce the risk of developing more serious health issues.

In conclusion, seeking professional help when needed is essential for individuals with gum disease. Dental professionals can provide the necessary treatment and guidance to help manage the condition and prevent it from worsening. By working closely with your dentist and following their recommendations, you can improve your oral health and reduce the risk of developing more serious health issues related to gum disease. Remember, your oral health is an important part of your overall wellbeing, so do not hesitate to seek help when needed.

How To Prevent Gum Disease

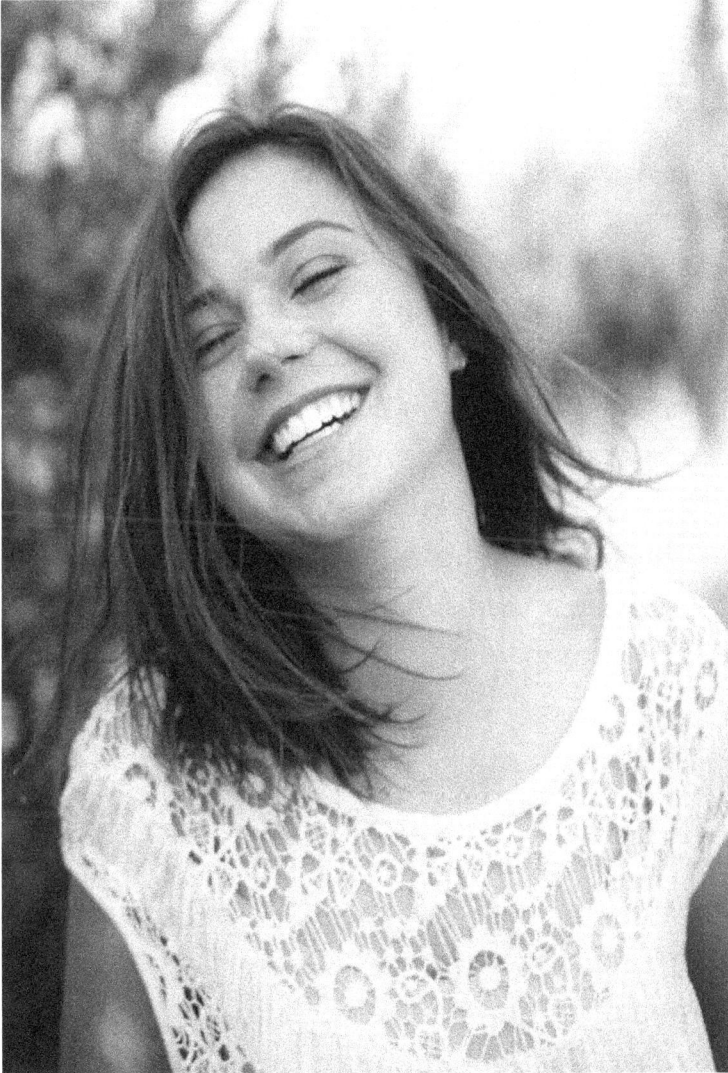

Chapter 9

Conclusion

Recap of Key Points

In this chapter, we have discussed the importance of preventing gum disease and maintaining good oral health. Gum disease, also known as periodontal disease, is a serious condition that can lead to tooth loss and other health complications if left untreated. It is caused by bacteria that build up on the teeth and gums, leading to inflammation and infection. By following a few simple steps, you can prevent gum disease and keep your mouth healthy.

First and foremost, it is essential to practice good oral hygiene habits. This includes brushing your teeth at least twice a day, flossing daily, and using mouthwash to kill bacteria. Proper brushing and flossing techniques are crucial for removing plaque and preventing gum disease. It is also important to visit your dentist regularly for check-ups and professional cleanings to ensure that any early signs of gum disease are detected and treated promptly.

Another key point to preventing gum disease is to avoid tobacco products. Smoking and chewing tobacco can increase your risk of developing gum disease and make it harder to treat. By quitting smoking and avoiding tobacco products, you can significantly improve your oral health and reduce your risk of gum disease.

Maintaining a healthy diet is also essential for preventing gum disease. Eating a balanced diet rich in fruits, vegetables, and whole grains can help strengthen your immune system and fight off bacteria that cause gum disease. Avoiding sugary and acidic foods and drinks can also prevent tooth decay and gum disease.

Overall, preventing gum disease requires a combination of good oral hygiene habits, regular dental visits, avoiding tobacco products, and maintaining a healthy diet. By following these key points, you can protect your gums and teeth from the damaging effects of gum disease and enjoy better oral health for years to come. Remember, prevention is always better than treatment when it comes to gum disease.

Final Tips for Preventing Gum Disease

As you continue on your journey to preventing gum disease, there are a few final tips that can help you maintain better oral health. One of the most important things you can do is to brush your teeth at least twice a day with a fluoride toothpaste.

This will help remove plaque and bacteria that can lead to gum disease. Make sure to brush gently and thoroughly, paying special attention to the gum line where bacteria tend to accumulate.

In addition to regular brushing, it is also important to floss daily. Flossing helps remove food particles and plaque from between your teeth, where your toothbrush cannot reach. This can help prevent gum disease and keep your gums healthy. If you have trouble flossing, consider using a water flosser or interdental brushes to clean between your teeth.

Another important tip for preventing gum disease is to visit your dentist regularly for check-ups and cleanings. Your dentist can help monitor the health of your gums and catch any signs of gum disease early on. They can also provide professional cleanings to remove plaque and tartar buildup that can contribute to gum disease.

By staying on top of your dental appointments, you can prevent gum disease from progressing and keep your smile healthy.

It is also important to maintain a healthy lifestyle to prevent gum disease. This includes eating a balanced diet, limiting sugary and acidic foods, and avoiding tobacco products. Smoking and using tobacco can increase your risk of gum disease and make it harder for your gums to heal. By making healthier choices and taking care of your overall health, you can reduce your risk of developing gum disease.

Lastly, be sure to pay attention to any changes in your gums, such as redness, swelling, or bleeding. If you notice any of these symptoms, make an appointment with your dentist right away. Early detection and treatment of gum disease can help prevent it from progressing and causing further damage to your oral health.

By following these final tips for preventing gum disease, you can take control of your oral health and enjoy a healthier smile for years to come.

Resources for Further Information

If you're looking for more information on preventing gum disease, there are plenty of resources available to help you learn more about this common oral health issue. One great place to start is the American Dental Association (ADA) website, which offers a wealth of information on gum disease, its causes, and how to prevent it. The ADA also provides tips on proper oral hygiene practices and the importance of regular dental check-ups in maintaining healthy gums.

Another valuable resource for individuals with gum disease is the National Institute of Dental and Craniofacial Research (NIDCR). This organization conducts research on oral health issues, including gum disease, and provides information on the latest advancements in prevention and treatment. The NIDCR website is a great place to find reliable information on the causes of gum disease, risk factors, and strategies for keeping your gums healthy.

For those looking for practical tips on preventing gum disease, the Mayo Clinic website is a great resource. The Mayo Clinic offers advice on maintaining good oral hygiene habits, including brushing and flossing techniques, as well as information on lifestyle factors that can impact gum health.

By following the recommendations on the Mayo Clinic website, you can take proactive steps to prevent gum disease and maintain a healthy smile.

How To Prevent Gum Disease

If you're interested in learning more about the connection between gum disease and overall health, the Centers for Disease Control and Prevention (CDC) website is a valuable resource. The CDC provides information on the links between gum disease and chronic conditions such as heart disease, diabetes, and respiratory problems.

By understanding the impact of gum disease on your overall health, you can take steps to prevent its progression and protect your well-being.

In addition to these online resources, don't hesitate to reach out to your dentist or dental hygienist for more information on preventing gum disease. These professionals are trained to assess your oral health and provide personalized recommendations for keeping your gums healthy. By taking advantage of the resources available to you, you can empower yourself to take control of your oral health and prevent gum disease before it becomes a serious issue.

Author Notes & Acknowledgments

First and foremost, I would like to express my deepest gratitude to the people who inspired and supported me throughout the journey of writing this book. This project would not have been possible without their unwavering belief in me and their invaluable contributions.

To my wife, thank you for your constant encouragement and understanding. Your love and support have been my anchor during the challenging times of researching and writing this book. Your belief in my ability to make a difference in people's lives has been my driving force.

I would also like to disclose that this book contains some renewed artificial intelligence-generated content. I really appreciate very recent technological innovation by outstanding scientists and of course our reader's understanding.

Lastly, I want to express my deepest gratitude to the readers of this book. I sincerely hope the strategies and methods outlined within these pages will provide you with the knowledge and tools needed to truly make your life much better. Your commitment to seeking any good solutions and willingness to explore multiple methods is commendable.

Author Bio

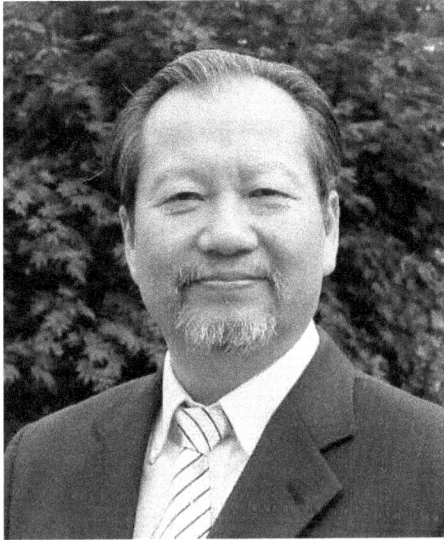

Johnson Wu earned his MD in 1982. With over 40 years of clinical experience, he has worked in hospitals in Zhejiang and Shanghai, China, as well as the Royal Marsden Hospital (part of Imperial College) in London, UK.

Upon the recommendation of Sir Aaron Klug, the president of The Royal Society and a Nobel Prize winner in Chemistry, Dr. Wu was honorably awarded a British Royal Society Fellowship. He has published medical books and articles in seven countries and currently practices medicine in Canada.

www.ingramcontent.com/pod-product-compliance
Lightning Source LLC
Chambersburg PA
CBHW060256030426
42335CB00014B/1724